Compassion in Nursing: Is It Necessary?

Compassion in Nursing: Is It Necessary?

Deborah J. Mauffray, RN, MSN, CNS, CWOCN

To order additional copies of this book, contact:
Xlibris Corporation
1-888-795-4274
www.Xlibris.com
Orders@Xlibris.com
65922

For the purpose of convenience, I used the female pronouns (she and her) when talking about nurses, unless I was telling a specific story that involved a male nurse. I used male pronouns (he/him) when discussing patients, unless I was telling a specific story about a female patient. Names in the book have been changed to protect individual privacy.

CHAPTER 1

Introduction

Imagine a dark hospital room with a 17 year-old girl sitting on the couch watching her aunt moan and groan in pain. It is the early 1970's, and the surgery her aunt had left her nose very swollen and looking like a large baked potato sitting on her face. The girl had already quietly and timidly stepped outside into the hallway to get the attention of a nurse. She knew her aunt needed pain medication. The girl had left the bathroom light on to give a little light, but otherwise the room was dark to allow her aunt to rest. Suddenly the door burst open, and the outline of a large-framed nurse came into the room. She walked over to her aunt's bed and flipped on the light without saying a word.

Then, in a sarcastic voice she said, "Did you need something for pain?" Before her aunt had a chance to even answer, the nurse flipped her over and stuck her in her left hip with a needle, before dropping her, unsupported, on her back once again. This took place in about five seconds total; or so it seemed to the girl who sat curled up in awestruck horror on the couch! Her aunt groaned as she was tussled from side to back to side, but she didn't say a word to the nurse. The girl was too afraid and naïve to say anything either.

That girl was me. My uncle had asked my parents if I could go stay with my aunt while she was in the hospital. She was going to be in a city about 50 miles away from home, and he had to work. My parents agreed, so there I was. Unlike today, during my school years, I was a very timid, quiet girl who would like to melt into the wood work and hope no one noticed I was there. I was a good student, but very shy. This was the summer between my junior and senior years in high school, and I was having trouble deciding which major I would choose for college. I grew up alternating between wanting to be a teacher one day and wanting to be a nurse the next. The catalyst that helped me make that final decision was when my paternal aunt, who happened to be a nurse, had to have surgery. The experience of watching that nurse with the white nurse's cap, white dress, white stockings and white shoes being rough, rude, and impatient was all it took to make my decision final. I decided right then and there I was going to become a nurse. And the main thing was I was going to be different than she.

I have been a nurse for over 32 years now, and I truly believe it was a calling from God. He put me . . . in *that* room . . . with *that* nurse . . . at *that* time in my life . . . so that I would make that choice. In all these years, I have witnessed other nurses with the same kind of attitude as that "Grinch," but I believe there are more nurses who are very compassionate people. This book is about compassion and nursing.

According to *The American Heritage Dictionary*, compassion is a noun that means a "deep awareness of the suffering of another coupled with the wish to relieve it." Nursing is a science as well as an art. The science has progressed a lot in the past three decades, such as new technology and new medications that have been developed over that time span. The art of nursing has more to do with the compassionate care by nurses. Any changes I have seen probably have to do with the life experiences of the nurses and the age differences of each graduating class every year or so. There are people who are going into nursing as a second career, so they are in nursing school in their thirties, forties or even older. Even with the variety of age, there are nurses, new graduates and experienced, who are immature. The immaturity can be evident in how they care for the patients.

For instance, as a wound care specialist, I was requested to see a patient for a wound on his shoulder. As was my custom, I reviewed the record to find out the patient's medical history, what had been documented related to the wound, and what the current wound care orders were. Then I went in to see the patient, assessed the wound, and decided what the wound care orders should be. After discussing this with the physician who had written the consult order, I then approached the nurse to discuss my findings with her. She informed me that the patient I had seen was going to surgery, and she didn't have time to talk to me. She was quick to tell me, also, that she knew everything she needed to know about him, and I didn't need to tell her anything. As it turned out, this was a new graduate nurse. I told the nurse preceptor assigned to her about my findings, instead. That "know-it-all" attitude is not real common, but it isn't rare, either. Some of the new nurses seem to come out of nursing school thinking they know everything.

In the book, *Through the Patient's Eyes: Understanding and Promoting Patient-Centered Care*, Gerteis, Edgman-Levitan, Daley and Delbanco (1993) compiled information about patients that were obtained from several national interviews related to their preferences for health care. One of the most mentioned ideas was that they need to feel like they are being cared for by competent (not overly confident) caregivers. It may just be me, but I don't generally trust someone who acts like they know everything—even doctors with many years experience—because nobody knows everything except God. When a patient asks me a question and I don't know the answer, I just tell him, "I don't know, but I'll try to find out and get back to you." The patient has much more respect for honesty rather than someone to make up an answer that might be wrong. I would rather be honest, at first, than have to go back and correct my misinformation.

As I watched this young nurse's career, it was obvious she really wasn't in nursing to care for patients. It seemed her objective was to bring home a paycheck. She was intelligent, but was impersonable, business-like in her attitude with her patients. She didn't stay at the hospital very long. I don't know where she went when she left, but I hope she found something she *loved* to do. I'm a firm believer that people should love their jobs. They should be happy with whatever kind of work they do, or they will probably be miserable. That may be an impossible thing to accomplish 100% of the time, but with nursing, there are way too many opportunities for people to find out if it's truly what they want to do.

There are many varieties of nursing jobs from which to choose once one becomes a nurse. One can work in a hospital in a variety of roles, or can work for a home health agency. Other occupations include working in an outpatient clinic, a doctor's office, nursing home, rehabilitation (rehab) facility and so on. In the hospital setting, one could work as a staff nurse, a manager, a patient educator or a staff educator, a clinical consultant, a case manager, quality nurse or infection control nurse. The opportunities are endless. The staff nurse can choose to take care of medical patients, surgical patients, cardiac patients, oncology patients, adult or children, in labor and delivery or post-partum, intensive care or emergency—the possibilities are multiple.

Nursing students can get jobs working as nursing techs or nursing assistants during school breaks and on weekends while they're in school. This gives them an opportunity to not only work with patients, but also work *around* and *with* other nurses to see what nursing is all about. One of the problems with students working with nurses is that it may have a negative effect on them. For example, if a student nurse happens to work with a nurse who isn't happy being a nurse, who doesn't *love* what she does, it can leave a negative impression on that student. Or on the other hand, it can have a positive effect. That student nurse may want to be a nurse even more, but be a better nurse than the one with whom she has been working.

John Townsend (2007) states that love is one of the things that guides our lives from beginning to end—how little or how much love we have affects us from cradle to grave. The Dalai Lama (2005) believes that the balance between the human brain and human compassion is lost, because we sometimes concentrate too much on our minds and neglect human affection or love. Sometimes we get so busy and involved in *doing* our job, that we don't take the time, or maybe we don't have the desire, to expend the energy to *demonstrate* the love. Nurses care. But care and love are not the same, and caring is not enough. To care means to be interested or concerned, to provide watchful supervision or needed assistance. To love means to experience deep affection for another. Another expression for love is "out of compassion; no thought for reward." Loving is relational. There has to be interaction with other people to develop loving relationships. Townsend (2007) identifies the key aspects of love as connecting (developing a bond), truth-telling (being honest), healing (repairing brokenness), letting go (surrendering things), and romancing (being a couple). The first four aspects of love should be evident in nursing. The last is a personal relationship with a spouse or fiancé. I am going to discuss the first four as how I believe they relate to nursing.

Connecting (developing an emotional bond):

When a nurse first meets a patient, a rapport should be developed. It doesn't have to be something that will be a lasting friendship, but something that gives the patient a feeling of confidence and assurance that he is in good hands. It may only last that particular visit, or continue a lifetime. On the negative side, getting too close to a patient and allowing that bond to go beyond a professional friendship can allow one to get too involved personally and emotionally. This can then carry over into the nurse's personal life. In the qualitative study Swanson (1990) performed which compared the responsibilities of parents, nurses, and physicians in caring for critically ill infants in a neonatal intensive care unit (NICU), one of her findings was that the compassion that one feels as a nurse can eventually turn into compassion fatigue. For example, she related a story of one nurse who became emotionally attached to an infant who eventually died. Because of that outcome (the infant's death), the nurse stepped away from direct care as the primary nurse of any infant and only assisted nurses in caring for their assigned patients to try to avoid getting caught up in that situation again. She stated she was "gun shy" and as soon as she felt like she was falling in love with one of the infants, she had to step back and let someone else take care of the patient so that she could take care of herself. Since the act of caring is to be concerned or interested and the act of loving is relational and is to experience a deep affection, then, to me, to care with love is compassion!

Truth-telling (honesty that serves the other person):

In nursing, this is one of the ethical principles that can make or break the trust between the patient and the health caregiver. With the availability of information, whether the accuracy is good or not, patients are better informed many times because they do research themselves or have someone else do the research. People don't like to be lied to and according to Drane (2002) in many cases it may be harmful to them. Trust is important to healing. If all possible interventions are not offered to the patients as choices, they lose their autonomy (independence). In this situation, the omission of complete information may lead to a sense of mistrust between the patient and the physician. What about nurses? How do we break the patients' trust by not telling the truth? When medications are given, if we don't teach the patients the name, dose, potential side effects, and what to report to the nurse or doctor, we are withholding information.

If we only tell patients part of the side effects list and not all (the more severe, for example), we are not telling the truth. If a patient needs to monitor his blood pressure, pulse or blood sugar, and we don't teach him how to do those things, we are withholding information that does not make him fully informed. That takes away his autonomy and ability to care for himself.

Drane agrees with Townsend by saying that human beings are relational, but where Townsend talks about loving relationships, Drane discusses truthful relationships. This is true for marital relationships as well as for relationships between doctors and patients and nurses and patients. Gerteis, et al (1993) identified that people want to be treated as individuals. Most patients desire to participate in their care, and they want honest, complete, and accurate information about their illness, prognosis and treatment options. Sometimes they may need help in making those decisions, and they rely on nurses to explain what has been told to them by the doctor. Bright, intelligent people can be ignorant to medical care, and it's very frightening when you're the one on the receiving end of that care. The patient may not know what questions to ask, but he wants the nurse to be able to provide answers. According to Gerteis, et al, communication was another component of nursing that indicates quality of healthcare. It is important to give the patient time to *hear* the information, *absorb* the information and then *process* the information given.

Healing (repairing brokenness):

Obviously, nurses put interventions that promote the healing process into practice. Nurses can play a huge role in providing assistance to patients who have things going on emotionally or, otherwise, that affects their physical well-being. For instance, a patient who is worried about his family, finances, job or whatever else that is interfering with his physical healing process can impact his physical well-being. A nurse who has a compassionate heart will be astute enough to pick up on little hints or comments made by the patient and spend an extra minute or two (even if she doesn't feel like she has it) to just talk to the patient—to let him know that he can talk about anything in which he wants. By listening, the nurse can collaborate with other healthcare providers such as social workers, case managers, etc., to possibly ease the patient's mind and help focus on his physical condition.

I've seen nurses who are so methodical and ritualistic—so organized—in their work that they do the tasks that have to be done without stopping to talk to the patient about anything other than the problem for which he is being treated. They don't stop and touch his hand or rub his forehead, or even give him comforting, reassuring words to say that they'll be back or will be close by if he's frightened or lonely. It's also well documented that it can be cost-effective to address patients' emotional needs. Some of the benefits to the patients who have that emotional support include leaving the hospital earlier, begin walking again more quickly, require less medication, comply more readily with treatment regimens, and experience fewer side effects from drugs. Because of these benefits, patients are more satisfied with their care. It is essential to provide emotional support to *all* patients if needed.

Letting Go (giving up what should be surrendered):

For some nurses this can be a difficult step in the nursing process. If they've developed a long-term relationship with a patient who is admitted into the hospital either actively dying or due to some unforeseen event, his heart stops, it may be difficult to withhold treatment and let go when the time comes. She usually does alright during the crisis; but after everything is calmed down and maybe after she's already gone home, it finally hits her. It has been shown that stress from continuously being faced with difficult family dynamics and multiple patients dying within a short period of time has a cumulative effect on nurses' coping abilities according to Abendroth and Flannery (2006). Eventually it can all catch up to them.

CHAPTER 2

In describing these key aspects of love, it is evident that nurses are in a profession, as other healthcare providers, that is high risk for burnout or compassion fatigue. A person's passion for his family, work, and activities provides meaning and value, but without love there is no satisfaction. As the apostle Paul said to the Corinthians, "And though I bestow all my goods to feed the poor and though I give my body to be burned, but have not love, it profits me nothing." I Corinthians 13:3 (*Life Application Study Bible*, NKJV, 1996). Townsend (2007) describes the benefits of becoming a loving person: 1) spiritual growth—love is the greatest gift given to us by God through His Son, Jesus, 2) better relationships—become better connected to family and friends, 3) quality of life—the positive effects of love may lead to better emotional and physical health according to some researchers, 4) the experience of love, 5) good effects of love on others—loving people empathize with, encourage and support others, 6) the capacity for intimacy—allows one's self to become connected to the hearts of others, 7) leadership abilities—inspire, motivate, and guide others to excel, 8) freedom—free to be one's own person, to make decisions and choices of his own, 9) personal growth and healing, 10) joy and happiness—contented, one receives more than he gives, 11) success in goals and dreams—loving people are enveloped in courage which helps them accomplish their visions, goals, and dreams. (pp. 6-8).

Burnout vs. Compassion Fatigue

Burnout is defined as physical or emotional exhaustion resulting from long term stress. Swanson (1990) defined it as the "loss of motivation for creative involvement." (p. 71) Either way, the causes or contributing factors of burnout may be: 1) an overloaded work schedule—that is, having too little time and too few resources to accomplish the job (Laschinger & Leiter, 2006), 2) spending too much time and energy trying to avoid bad outcomes, and 3) continual management of responsibilities. These factors tend to take the place of spending time caring and attaching to the patient, which are rewarding and energizing (Swanson, 1990). Also, when the care provided by the nurse is evaluated only by how well she avoided errors and managed responsibilities, the roles of caring and attaching are ignored, or in my case, reprimanded.

I remember learning in nursing school that "you should never get too close to the patient." "Don't show emotion around the family." That's very hard to do. When I was working in ICU, there was an elderly woman who was the matriarch of a very large family. There were children, grandchildren and great-grandchildren in the waiting room. At that time the youngest visitor allowed was 12 years old and it was a small waiting room! I was the charge nurse that day and visiting hours were pretty strict. Only two visitors at a time could go in the patient's room for ten minutes every two hours. This woman was dying, and the family was desperate to see her before she died. I broke the rules and allowed more than two family members to go in if they agreed to stay only a few minutes so that all members would have a chance to visit. They agreed and were very appreciative. By mid-day, all of the family had been given a chance to see her and say their goodbyes. It was a very emotional time, and I shed quite a few tears with quite a few of the family members.

There were other patients' families who got upset when I wouldn't let them visit their loved one in the same fashion. But, when I explained what was going on, they were very cooperative and understanding.

When it came time for my evaluation, I was reprimanded on paper for being "too emotional" around the patients, and he cited that incident. He wasn't even there; he just heard about it. I believe the family totally disagreed with him. They appreciated the sincerity and compassion. After all, Jesus wept when he knew that Lazarus had died.

The side effects of burnout include pessimism, fatalism, depression, hopelessness, and apathy. All of these can be self-perpetuating. Burnout occurs slowly and is the result of long-term work-related issues and can occur in any general population, not just in health care.

At the conclusion of the article by Swanson (1990), she shared one of the parent's responses to the interviews that were done regarding the caring phenomenon. The parent described what happens in the NICU everyday in one phrase as being an act of love.

> An act of love is what it is, you, there is no other way to describe it. 'Cause those people in there, they work so hard. I've talked to the nurses about it, about having so many babies come in and out of their lives and the emotional attachments they make. You know there's a lot of emotions in there. There's the mother, the father, the nurses, the doctors. I'd have to say an act of love more than anything else. On everybody's part.

On my part, being there, love for my son. And he got here, I had him because I *wanted* to have him and I definitely felt something for him. I'd have to say that would be it. On the whole, the NICU, you wanted a phrase that would get it all, I'd have to say it was an act of love (p. 72).

Compassion fatigue is different than burnout in that it is specific to professions who choose to help others. It is defined as an emotional drain experienced by caregivers usually after caring for another with a progressive illness. It is usually a rapid onset problem and can be related to one particular event or long-term exposure to many traumatic stories or events. This was really evident after Hurricane Katrina on the Mississippi Gulf Coast (and I'm sure the Louisiana Gulf Coast area also). Nurses were taking care of people who had survived the worst natural disaster to ever hit that region since Hurricane Camille. Some had thought they would never live to see another storm like Camille, and had now lived through a storm which was possibly even worse. The problem was that many of the nurses and other healthcare providers had experienced the same kind of loss the patients had experienced, and they were having to listen to everyone else's stories over . . . and over . . . and over again . . . without having the opportunity to tell their own story. Many wouldn't even tell their co-workers or friends about their losses because they knew they were in the same situation.

Nurses left the area. Nurses left nursing. Nurses began exhibiting the symptoms of compassion fatigue. Those symptoms include: difficulty sleeping, increased startle response, avoidance of places or things that are reminders of the event(s), obtrusive thoughts and images about the event(s), and depressed and/or anxious mood. Job-specific causes of compassion fatigue include: long exposure to the suffering of others, patient death, little to no emotional support in the workplace, inadequate preparation, conflict with co-workers (Alkema, Linton, and Davies, 2008, Radley & Figley cited in Alkema, et al, 2008). Others include stress, listening to descriptions of traumatic events experienced by others, anxiety, life demands, and excessive empathy (leading to blurred professional boundaries) (Abendroth & Flannery, 2006), and poor self-care (Radley & Figley cited in Alkema, et al, 2008). Nurses who are inclined to put their patients' needs ahead of their own may also be prone to paying attention to their own needs last in other areas of their lives.

A few weeks after Hurricane Katrina hit land, one of the local hospitals on the Mississippi Gulf Coast invited its staff to "tell their stories" in front of a film crew. This was an effort to counter the effects the storm was having on the staff. It proved to be very therapeutic for many of them. Not only were they able to tell what happened to them personally before, during and after the storm, but they got to share what had transpired since that time. Some staff focused on personal trials, and others shared their experiences in the hospital. But, nonetheless, it seemed to be helpful to the ones who participated.

The dictionary doesn't define the "caregiver" specifically as professionals. So compassion fatigue may occur when someone is caring for a loved one for long periods of time without breaks or ways of performing self-care activities, whether it's going shopping, getting her hair done or walking on the beach while someone else is providing the care for the person who is ill or confined to the home. The study that Alkema, et al (2008) performed was to investigate whether the healthcare providers who participated in several self-care activities would experience higher levels of compassion satisfaction and lower levels of compassion fatigue and burnout. (Compassion satisfaction is gratification resulting from the efforts of one's labors.) The results suggested that emotional and spiritual self-care activities and personal-professional balance are predictive of higher levels of compassion satisfaction as compared to physical, psychological and workplace areas of activities.

Rohan and Bausch (2009) describe the roles of physicians, social workers and nurses, delineate the roles among the professions, and then describe how the roles complement each other. This is very much like the body of Christ.

> "For as the body is one and has many members, but all the members of that one body, being many, are one body, so also is Christ. . . . . If the foot should say, 'Because I am not a hand, I am not of the body,' is it therefore not of the body? And if the ear should say, 'Because I am not an eye, I am not of the body, Is it therefore not of the body? If the whole body were an eye, where would be the hearing? If the whole were hearing, where would be the smelling? But now God has set the members, each one of them, in the body just as He pleased. And if they were all one member, where would the body be?
>
> But now indeed there are many members, yet one body. And the eye cannot say to the hand, 'I have no need of you'; nor again the head to the feet, 'I have no need of you.' No, much rather, those members of the body which seem to be weaker are necessary. And those members of the body which we think to be less honorable, on these we bestow greater honor;

and our unpresentable parts have greater modesty, but our presentable parts have no need. But God composed the body, having given greater honor to that part which lacks it, that there should be no schism in the body, but that the members should have the same care for one another. And if one member suffers, all the members suffer with it; or if one member is honored, all the members rejoice with it." I Corinthians 12:12, 15-25, (*Life Application Study Bible*, NKJV, 1996).

Just like it takes all parts of the body to make a whole, it takes the whole healthcare team to provide the care necessary for compassionate care. Rohan and Bausch studied the population of groups of healthcare providers which worked with oncology patients. The authors described symptoms of professional grief that occurred when the staff experienced repeated relationships that ended in death. The symptoms included helplessness, depression, boredom, apathy, guilt, displaced anger, work-related dreams, withdrawal from their dying patient and questioning of values of the work. They may also encounter anxiety, uncertainty, and may have strong reactions to the sights, smells, and sounds of cancer (Rohan & Bausch, 2009).

Some go home every night and cry about a patient, others have anxiety attacks. Still others have psychosomatic afflictions and post-traumatic stress disorder (PTSD) symptoms at some points during their careers. Some have dreams of patients, dream of themselves dying, or have thoughts of specific details of their own funerals.

In the study, to endure and replenish themselves, some of the activities in which the healthcare providers participated included: exercising, pursuing hobbies, taking vacations, reconnecting with nature, focusing on family, talking with family or friends, seeking refuge, engaging in spiritual practices and other rituals when patients die (such as going to their funerals), adjusting their expectations of success, and perceiving their work differently over time. Some reorganize career or work priorities to reflect more balance by working in a less clinically intense position, reducing work hours, or working in research.

I have experienced compassion fatigue personally myself. It happened after I spent five weeks taking care of my father as he was dying from acute lymphocytic leukemia with metastasis to his liver and renal cell carcinoma. My mother was hospitalized for a week during that time for a heart catheterization, and my sister had to work the first three weeks. She worked the night shift so she would try to sleep during the day. My husband was at our home taking care of his father who had recently had an amputation of one of his legs. This left me by myself taking care of Daddy who was confused and disoriented because of the cancer that had spread to his brain. He was weak but when he tried to get out of the bed (climbing over side rails) or wanted to "use the bathroom," he would fight every step of the way while I was trying to help him. He was as strong as an ox then! Daddy never did remember my name—he called everyone else by name, but me. That may not seem important to anyone else, but it still haunts me to this day and it's been five years since he passed away.

I loved Daddy and still do. It was one of the hardest things in my entire nursing career to do—to watch my daddy die. I had seen many people die in my career, and several family members, but nothing touched me as personally as being there with my daddy. No matter how much anyone consoled me, it didn't seem to help. After he died and we went through the funeral service, my family and I went on a trip for me to "get away" from the memories of the past few weeks. I thought that would help me recuperate and help me get back to work refreshed.

As it turned out, when I went back to work, things started falling apart. I am a specialty nurse and the types of patients I specialize in caring for are those who have stomas of some kind. They may have a colostomy, ileostomy or urostomy. These are surgical procedures where the bodily function of emptying the bowels or bladder has been redirected to come out through an opening in the side of the patient's abdomen. I also specialize in wound care and skin problems associated with stomas and wounds. As part of my job, I receive consults from physicians and nurses to treat these problems, and to assist patients with learning how to handle themselves at home.

During my time with Daddy, there was no one available to assist these patients except the staff nurses who don't have the specialized training that I have. They did their best, but some of the patients had to be seen by me as outpatients to help them with problems that could have been prevented if I had been there to take care of them. I took this realization very personally. There was one patient currently in the hospital when I came back from funeral leave who had a problem ileostomy. The nurses had been changing her ostomy appliance (what collected the stool) very frequently and her skin was very irritated to the point of burns on her abdomen. I blamed myself for this even though I wasn't to blame—"I should have taught the nurses how to manage it better" or "I shouldn't have taken off that extra time after Daddy died" or "why didn't someone else know how to fix this problem?" were all thoughts that went through my head.

The patient was very appreciative of my attention and, with time, her skin healed and she learned how to manage her ostomy. But unfortunately, I was getting worse about feeling responsible every time one of my patients had a problem. I started losing weight, having female problems, developed irritable bowel syndrome, and my migraines that had been controlled got worse. I had several episodes of transient ischemic attacks where I had weakness on one side of my body and inability to talk clearly. Then finally one day, I was in a grocery store with my husband and had a focal seizure which resulted in me being sent to the hospital. The stress had caught up with me, and I had to learn some major lessons. If it weren't for God being with me every step of the way during that time, I don't know what would have happened to me. I became very depressed and had feelings of being unworthy. My family, friends and church family were all trying to be supportive, and I'm sure they were praying for me (which is what sustained me). But I couldn't get Daddy's death out of my mind, and I was trying too hard to please everyone else.

Eventually, after multiple trips to physicians' offices, being put on anti-depressant medications, and having surgery that gave me time off, I finally came to the realization that I can't "fix" all problems. I realized that I will not be available for every patient all the time, especially if I am sick myself, or worse yet, dead. It took time, but I actually began feeling like I was being used by patients. I felt like I was being used without positive feedback from them. I got the feedback from other healthcare providers, but not from the patients. That was not like me at all. Usually I love what I do and am very grateful to God that He gave me the opportunity to work in the nursing field in which I have been blessed to serve. The compassion fatigue had hit me like a train barreling across the railroad tracks at 70 miles per hour!

I eventually changed jobs. It was not until I decided to write this book, and began doing the research for it that I discovered exactly what compassion fatigue is all about. I lived it! I was beginning to think that there are very few nurses who really enjoy nursing. I thought there are some people who are in nursing for what they can get out of it—and it isn't the rewards of seeing sick people get better. I still believe there are some in nursing like that, but now I believe that there are many more who do love their jobs. But, as what was mentioned numerous times in the many articles I read, listening to other people's problems and dealing with life and death situations day in and day out can become more of a trial than it is worth after a while. The results of my survey, small as it was, still found that the respondents rated the level of compassionate care to be 5.5 out of 7. This is pretty good when one of the outliers was a two and one was a seven. We all could use more compassion at times, and I believe that as nurses, we need to do a better job at separating ourselves from the everyday struggles we hear about when we are at work.

Watson (1999) remarks, "We recognize that, even though medicine and other health professions throughout time have been based upon a philosophy of caring and healing, we find ourselves at the end of the 20th century having to make a case for caring and healing." Are nurses still compassionate? Yes, there is still compassion in nursing. But in my experiences of observing the nursing profession over the past 32 years, it seems to me that there seems to be fewer "called," and more going into nursing for different reasons. This, I believe, is impacting the caring-healing of the patient and the family unit. As Schultz (1987) advised, the patient is more than just the patient. The family, which may include close friends, is to whom the care is provided.

There are not always negative results of taking care of sick or dying patients. Rohan and Bausch (2009) identified rewards of working with oncology patients as: being able to ease suffering, receiving gratitude from patients, having intimate emotional connections with patients, being inspired and awed by the human spirit, and gaining wisdom and perspective. This could carry over to all patients, not just oncology patients. Most clinicians who work with dying patients who had regrets found that the patient's regrets were never about work; they were always about relationships. People spoke of wishing they hadn't missed their children's dance recitals, school plays, or sports games. They never spoke of wishing for one last promotion at work. We should learn from them.

CHAPTER 3

The Survey

I conducted a survey in which I sent out 75 questionnaires (see Appendix A). I had two objectives: 1) to find out what kinds of personal experiences, if any, the individual responding may have had with healthcare providers, especially nurses, and 2) to obtain stories they may want to share with me regarding those experiences. The questionnaire included questions about whether the person had been in a hospital, nursing home, had home health or been in an inpatient rehabilitation personally. There was also a question to find out if any of them had a family member in either of those settings. And finally, did any of the respondents know anyone else personally in either of those settings. I did this because there are people who have not experienced inpatient care themselves but they have probably witnessed the care of someone they love or know in their lifetime.

I also wanted to see if the people responding had a good grasp of the difference between sympathy, empathy and compassion. To do that, I added a question regarding the definition of compassion using the definitions of the other two words as two of the choices.

Another part of the survey was to determine where the respondents ranked the nurses in how compassionate they were in providing care. A Likert scale ranging from 1-7 was used, with one being "no compassion at all," four being "neutral" and seven being "demonstrated great compassion." Then I asked them for their opinion of which of the following list of nursing activities indicates that a nurse is compassionate: a) plans quality time with the patient, b) actively listens to the patient, c) always presents with a caring attitude, d) keeps promises, e) keeps patient informed of changes, f) problem solves to resolve patient concerns, g) involves patient in plan of care, h) involves family in plan of care when appropriate, and i) provides dignity and respect to the patient. Finally, I asked them to write one or more stories of personal experiences they had related to the compassionate care or lack of compassion they may have experienced.

I distributed a total of 75 questionnaires. Some were mailed randomly selecting names from the phone book. I left some in my church for the members to anonymously respond it they chose to, and I gave some to my co-workers. There was a return of 13 surveys, which was a 17 percent return rate. There were ten female (77%) and three male (23%) respondents, and 100% of them had been a patient in a hospital at some point in their lives. One of them had also received home health personally. Twelve of the thirteen (92%) had had a loved one in a hospital in the past. Fifty-four percent had a loved one in a nursing home, 38% had a loved one who received home health and eight percent had a loved one in an inpatient rehab facility in the past. See Table 1 for the percentage of people who had known someone other than family (e.g., friends) who had been in either of the settings.

	Personally a Patient	Family a Patient	Friend a Patient
Hospital	100%	92%	77%
Nursing Home		54%	38%
Home Health	8%	38%	31%
IP Rehab		8%	23%

Table 1

Interestingly, the nursing activities that were found to be most important as it relates to compassion in the opinions of the survey respondents were right in alignment with the national study in which Gerteis, et al (1993) discusses patient-centered care. The top two activities both received 83% of the votes (see Table 2). They were 1) actively listens to the patient and 2) provides dignity and respect to patient/family. The next highest activity came in at 75% and was: keeps patient informed of changes. Sixty-seven percent of the votes were given to the next three activities: 1) problem-solves to resolve patient concerns, 2) involves patient in the plan of care, and 3) involves family in plan of care when possible. The fourth activity, at 58%, was: always presents with a caring attitude. Finally the lowest ranked activities were keeps promises at 50% and plans quality time with patient at 42% (See Table 2).

	Percentage
Quality time	42%
Actively listens	83%
Caring attitude	58%
Keeps promises	50%
Keeps informed	75%
Problem solves	67%
Involves patient	67%
Involves family	67%
Dignity & respect	83%

Table 2

The seven primary dimensions of patient-centered care as described in Gerteis et al (1993) are:

1. Respect for patients' values, preferences and expressed needs (quality of life, involvement in decision making, dignity, needs and autonomy)
2. Coordination and integration of care (coordination and integration of clinical care, coordination and integration of ancillary and support services, coordination and integration of "front-line" patient care)
3. Information, communication and education (information on clinical status, progress, and prognosis, information on processes of care, information and education to facilitate autonomy, self-care and health promotion)
4. Physical comfort (pain management, help with activities of daily living, surroundings and hospital environment)
5. Emotional support and alleviations of fear and anxiety (anxiety over clinical status, treatment, and prognosis, anxiety over the impact of the illness on self and family, anxiety over the financial impact of the illness)

6. Involvement of family and friends (accommodation of family and friends, involving family in decision making, supporting the family as caregiver, recognizing the needs of the family)
7. Transition and continuity (information, coordination and planning, support) (pp. 5-11).

As identified in the survey, the things that the respondents desired most are included in the above list. Patient-centered care is just what it says—patient centered. When a nurse assigns a patient to get his bath at 10:00 in the morning because that's when there is enough staff to do it, that is not patient-centered; that is nurse-centered care. Especially if that patient prefers taking baths or showers in the evening. When a nurse wakes a patient up to do a procedure because that is the time she is available, that is not patient-centered care. The respondents in my survey rated the nurses' level of compassionate care to be 5.5 on a 1-7 scale, which is above average. When one compares that response to the stories they shared, that score seems high. Apparently, despite the evidence of lack of compassion, there was more evidence of true compassion.

CHAPTER 4

Stories from Survey:

As part of the survey I performed, one of the requests I had was that the respondents share a story related to compassion that was experienced personally. In the following pages, I am going to share the stories that were submitted in the questionnaires that were returned. Some of the stories I obtained through interviews with family and friends and were not part of the survey, but the stories are significant just the same. Most are quoted verbatim. One is paraphrased, but you will get the intent of the story.

Tess' story:

"I think that compassionate nursing requires a nurse to be satisfied with [her] life and how [she is] treated as an individual by others. The golden rule—'do unto others as you would have them do unto you' is certainly a part of this type of person. My most recent experience with compassionate care was when my grandmother was hospitalized and 'suffered a massive brainstem stroke.' At least that was what the learned physician stated as he condemned my grandmother to a nursing home. He was the worst form of non-compassionate professionalism that I know, and of course the nurses followed suit by frowning and sighing at me as I refused to allow my grandmother to be ignored or labeled a 'no code [do not resuscitate].' My aunts had agreed to this label before I got to the bedside, having to travel to reach her. One look and I knew that this was all a game, a write-off for a woman who spent all her life raising children, scolding grandchildren and teaching them at the same time to do the right thing (we were supposed to be outside and not under her feet). She also taught me to bake, curl her hair and to feel a wonderful warmness when I rubbed her soft arms (she hated this as she thought I was playing with her 'fat'). Anyway—I wasn't going to let it happen and had the ability to do something. A couple of days and a neurologist consult later, my grandmother 'woke up' to the astonishment of her children and the nurses. All she needed was an antibiotic appropriate for her urosepsis [urinary tract infection]. Along the way, I did get to meet several nursing assistants and nurses, who did give the family a chance, gave them the time to grieve and the time to hope and for those nurses I was grateful. My grandmother did eventually die—about 6 months later, at home with hospice care and with dignity. A victim of a failing heart, too many co-morbidities [health problems]—but all of her 12 children, countless grandchildren and great-grandchildren were able to reconcile, gather around her, celebrate her last birthday and rub those soft arms before she passed away. The hospice nurses were wonderful; provided all the love and support as well as technical expertise that my family needed at that point—and I could then let her go too."

Tess' story gives us an example of how some nurses follow a physician's lead instead of being a patient or family advocate. This betrays two of the seven primary dimensions of patient-centered care that people desire—1) respect for patient's values, preference, and expressed needs, and 2) involvement of family (Gerteis, et al, 1993). Neither the physician nor the nurses were "listening" to Tess' requests. As it turned out, the first diagnosis was wrong and the treatment ended up being simple, comparatively speaking. Her grandmother's quality of life was much improved, and her family had time to spend with her prior to her death.

Tess used the Golden Rule as a guide for nursing—"And just as you want men to do to you, you also do to them likewise." Luke 6:31 (*Life Application Study Bible*, NKJV, 1996). Nurses are in a good position to exemplify this on a daily basis. I've often encouraged nurses to treat their patients the way they would want to be treated or they would want their mother to be treated.

Betsy's story:

Betsy's husband, Sam, was diagnosed with cancer May 7, 2004. She had experiences with nurses who cared, and those who did not care. Sam had to have surgery to laser through a tumor in the left bronchus, so the doctors would be able to proceed with a brain surgery that was needed. Following the successful surgery, he developed complications afterward. She was allowed to go into the unit he was in and she discovered he was in a lot of distress. He could not breathe, so he was sitting up fighting the nursing staff. There was a perforation that did not allow him to breathe even though he was intubated (had a tube in his throat to help him breathe). Betsy tried to tell the nurses he couldn't breathe and one particular nurse stated, "He is intubated. He is getting all the air he needs." Betsy looked at Sam and asked if he was able to breathe. He shook his head "no" with tears running down his face. His face had begun to swell so much one could no longer see his ears. His chest was also swelling which was indicative of air going where it should not have been. The doctor was rushing around trying to handle the situation. She told the nurse that she needed to help him. The nurse proceeded to speak rudely, and told Betsy that she did not know what was going on, and that he was fine. At that time, the nurse did not know that Betsy was a nurse. When the doctor informed the nurse that she was a nurse, the nurse said she did not need anyone to tell her how to observe and handle her patient. At that point the doctor had the nurse removed.

A week later, he was admitted to another hospital to have his brain surgery. The surgery was to remove an abscess that had developed in the cerebellum that was compressing the pons unit. This surgery was also successful, but once again, he developed complications. He hemorrhaged after the surgery and they had to reenter the surgical site. At this time, she and her family were told that what was thought to be an abscess was really a malignant tumor. He was admitted to the intensive care unit (ICU), but the nurses were so different from the previous week. The nurses were very nice and considerate to her and all the family. They would allow her to remain with Sam even after visiting hours were over, and they allowed her to help with his activities of daily living. If they needed her to leave, they would call her back in when they were finished with what they had to do. They offered her snacks and drinks and anything she needed. They were wonderful with the care of her husband and her.

Starting July 2, 2004, Sam began developing complications from his cancer. He was admitted to a third facility for dehydration and pneumonia. He was in the hospital for two days during this visit and was treated wonderfully. Once again, he had nurses that provided them with what they needed, but also gave them time together as he was able to still take care of himself. During this time, he was also receiving chemotherapy and radiation treatments.

Eight days after his discharge, he was admitted again to the third facility because of fever, not eating well, and difficulty with chemotherapy and radiation. He was on the same unit as before and had several of the same nurses. But there were some nurses who were not very caring. Sam's mediport (a device implanted under the skin that allows access to a blood vessel for infusing medication and/or fluids) was infected. He kept complaining of pain in the area of the mediport, and when Betsy pulled back the gauze, she checked for elevated temperature around the site. The site was swollen, reddened, hot, and when she barely pressed to feel the heat of the area, pus starting coming out of the site. She immediately went to the nurses' station and asked someone to go check it. The nurse went into the room and saw exactly what Betsy was talking about. She told Betsy that it was normal for this to happen, and that she would tell the doctor about it when he came in. Once again, she did not divulge her background so they were unaware of her knowledge. She proceeded to clean up the site, so the nurse brought her bandages to do it. The nurse was not going to clean the area, and she told Betsy it would be good practice for her, since she would need to take care of it at home. Betsy called the doctor and informed him of the problem. Within the hour, he had made arrangements for Sam to have his mediport removed that day. The doctor was not very happy with the way this nurse handled the problem, nor with the things that she said to Betsy. Once the mediport was removed, Sam began to feel better, and they were on their way home again. The nurse was reassigned to another unit after this event.

On August 24, 2004, Betsy went to pick up Sam from a hotel where his sister was staying. He had stayed to visit with her overnight since she was going back home to California that day. When Betsy picked him up, he was drenched with sweat and was burning up. They returned to the emergency department of the third facility again and he was taken immediately back to a room. The doctor went in and did his assessment. When the doctor came back, he called Betsy out of the room, and he had a nurse with him. As she went out of the room, Sam yelled out to her to hurry back; they had to make vacation plans. She started laughing because Sam was always a jokester. Little did she know that she was about to get hit with the ultimate question—"What do you want his code status to be?" She literally felt her body "faint without actually passing out." The nurse was there to make sure she didn't fall and offered her a drink, a chair, and a quiet place to talk to her or a chaplain if she needed. Betsy was really thankful that she was there at that moment.

The doctor then told her that she should call all the family in for probably the last time. His sister was there and they discussed the situation. Betsy and Sam had discussed what he desired to be done if he became unable to make decisions for himself. All his wishes were written down for her and she followed them as he wanted. That was the hardest thing for her to do, even though she knew that Sam did not want to be resuscitated if he stopped breathing or his heart stopped. To say those words and make that choice for him was heart-wrenching for her. The nurse stayed with her, and offered to make calls while she dealt with this trial. Sam was admitted to the hospital, and this would be for the last time.

Once they were admitted to the inpatient unit, the nurses there were wonderful once again. Betsy stayed at the hospital with Sam twenty-four hours a day, seven days a week. They allowed her to take care of him. She did everything for him except give him his medications. She turned him, bathed him, fed him when he was able to eat, read to him, and did anything she could to make him comfortable. The nurses even went the extra mile and had meals ordered for her. Several days into his stay, he began to go in and out of consciousness. She knew it was getting close, but she also knew Sam was waiting for her to let him go. She asked all the family to go in the room, and to talk to him. After that was done, Sam perked up and actually woke up. He was just like the man she knew before this illness was diagnosed. It was wonderful to see him as "his old self." He was awake for two days and then went back into an unconscious state. She slept next to him and held his hand every moment she could.

On Monday, September 6, Labor Day, the doctor came in and said that Sam would not be leaving the hospital alive. Since all the family was in the room, she went out into the hall with him, and asked him what his thoughts were. He said, "Probably tonight he will go." She lost all control in her legs and went down to the floor. The nurse ran over to her and escorted her to an empty room. She sat with Betsy while her tears ran down her cheeks. She was trying so hard to be strong for her family and knew she had to compose herself. The nurse starts crying with her and told Betsy she was there for her. She even gave her cellular phone number so Betsy could call her if she needed to talk to someone. She knew that nurses should not do that but she felt connected with her.

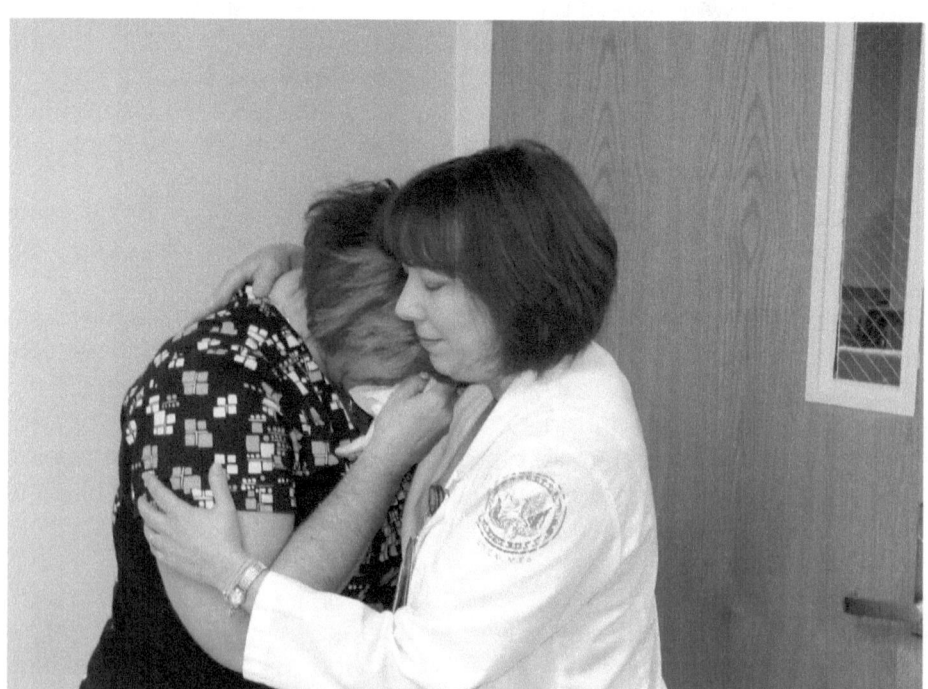

After some time, she returned to her husband and family. Everyone left to have dinner and to take a break. Betsy refused to leave the room. While she was alone with him, she told him that she was being selfish and did not want him to leave. She told him how much she loved him, and that she always would love him. She told him that she understood, and that she did not want him to suffer anymore. That they would be ok and that she would always know he was with her. She told him it was time for him to be released from all this pain, and that there were many children with God in which he needed to help. Sam had dedicated his life to youth and volunteered with youth events such as sports, etc. He was well loved.

Out of nowhere, she heard his voice telling her, "I love you." The tears were bittersweet—joy for hearing those words which she would always have and sorrow because she knew it would be the last time.

The nurses kept a constant check on her while she stayed with Sam. She would not leave his side. They took a collection and ordered pizza for her, because they had watched her not eating. Several of them went in the room, and they ate with Betsy. They talked about life and good times. Those few minutes with those nurses meant so much to her, as it gave her a break to let her emotions unwind a little. Her family started coming back, and they went back to their vigil. The next morning she was holding Sam's hand, and he took a deep breath. She checked him. That was his last breath. She went out to the hall, and looked at the far end of the hall. There was the nurse who had helped her so much. The nurse knew by the look on Betsy's face that the time had come. She rushed down to her and went into the room to check Sam. He was pronounced deceased on September 7, 2004, only a little more than three months from the time he was diagnosed. After his death, the nurses were very warm and caring to her. One nurse even prayed with her. It takes very special nurses to be able to deal with these situations on a daily basis. She said she will always be grateful to the nurses who helped take care of her while she worried about Sam.

Betsy described both negative and positive interactions with nurses. She was living through a difficult time in her life and needed what most people need—the confirmation that her loved one was being provided the best care possible, but also provided with compassion. This story makes me wonder if there would be fewer law suits if nurses, or any healthcare provider, would show more compassion when confronted with real issues rather than shrug them off. Because Betsy was a nurse, she knew what to expect. Because of the internet, many people are better informed than they used to be. They don't have to be nurses to be informed.

Davidson (2009) did a literature review related to the care of families who had loved ones in a critical care setting. It was established that one of the largest volume of complaints offered by patients' families related to restricted access to their loved ones and poor communication. As described in Betsy's story, when she was allowed to stay with Sam, she felt the compassion and caring from the staff. When the nurses failed to respond to her requests, such as when he was having difficulty breathing or when his mediport was infected, she felt the nurses weren't caring or compassionate.

Davidson (2009) also shared the findings from other research that nurses repeatedly underestimate the importance of a family's needs, such as the need for information or the need to be close to the patient. Nurses tend to make presumptions about the family's needs, and develop interventions around those presumptions rather than ask the family. Two additional needs identified are the need to provide support and the need to protect the patient. Research has shown that the psychological impact of critical illness on a patient's family member includes increased risk for anxiety, depression and post-traumatic stress disorder (PTSD).

Vernon's Story:

"My mother was in the hospital. She had been in there for several days. The staff was as nice and outpouring as you could be. Then one morning my twin brother got to the hospital before me and he overheard my mother's nurse down the hallway, while he is standing in her doorway, saying that she was 'tired of taking care of all of these old women.' The problem I had with that, she was saying it on the floor so most of the patients could hear it and most of the nurses, too. When I got to the hospital, I asked him if she had been in our mother's room. He said, 'Yes.' My comment was, 'Too bad.' Little did he know [but] my wife was a nurse and went straight to her supervisor. I told the supervisor what the nurse had said and that I didn't think the other patients would appreciate her comments either. I didn't see her anymore after that. I think she was burned out and really needed a change or time off."

Vernon's perception of how his mother's nurse was acting reminds me of the lack of two of the key aspects of love—connecting and truth-telling. The nurse definitely didn't "connect" with his mother's family by saying the things she did. There was also distrust by the family after the nurse made the derogatory comment. The rest of the nurses were compassionate and caring it seems, but the majority of his story was about the negative attitude of the one nurse. Like it is said, it takes nine positive comments or actions to counteract one negative.

Fran's Story:

"My mother [was] in the last stage of COPD and CHF. The nurses attending were not concerned with her pain control. The nurses in the hospital were not supportive during the family's distress. The physician finally called Hospice to help. The Hospice nurse was a life saver. He attended to my mother's pain and the families' needs. He gave my mother a dignified death at home with her family. The nursing staff had one nurse (who worked in the ICU) out of 10-12 nurses during her seven days stay in the hospital that was compassionate and caring—1 out of 10-12 cared."

This lady had a very negative experience at the hospital due to the poor pain management of her mother. Controlling pain was one of the most important requirements of medical care mentioned in the survey done related to patient-centered care by Gerteis, et al (1993). We have been told that pain is the fifth vital sign and yet pain management is still a problem in the hospital setting. The hospice staff have it mastered, it seems. She was very positive about how he (the hospice nurse) met her mother's and the family's needs. Unfortunately, only one out of 10-12 of the hospital nurses was compassionate and caring from her perception. "But You, O Lord, are a God full of compassion, and gracious, longsuffering and abundant in mercy and truth." Psalm 86:15 (*Life Application Study Bible*, NKJV, 1996).

Lilly's Story:

"I was blessed with a husband for forty-nine years. He was a well man most of his life. In 2005-2006 he was in and out of a [local hospital] about 12 times. Each time we were there, I have to say we were given real good care by all nurses and doctors. The nurses would come in and inform us to any changes the doctors ordered or if they were going to do tests. Before this time, when my husband had neck surgery in Feb 2006, we were at [another local hospital]. Our experience there before and after surgery wasn't pleasing as we were not informed by the doctor as to how my husband did after surgery! Three weeks after surgery he developed CHF [congestive heart failure], COPD [chronic obstructive pulmonary disease] and lung problems. He was never well again! God called him home August 17th, 2007. I give God the praise for not letting him suffer any longer!"

This is another story that relates to communication and the importance of sharing information. Lilly had experiences on both ends of the spectrum, and was much happier with the staff that informed and communicated.

Manny's Story:

"During my most recent stay at a VA medical facility the nurses that waited on me were very considerate of my limitations and pain. They made sure that I had assistance when getting in and out of bed. After my recovery and I was placed in a room it was late that night and the nurse took time to find me a meal to eat and that really impressed me due to the fact it was so late that night."

By taking that extra time and going out of their way to find a meal after hours—those actions were as important as the technical aspects of care, according to the survey compiled by Gerteis, et al (1993). There were 82% of the ones interviewed in that national survey who reported that someone went that extra mile to make their hospital stay more comfortable. Eighty-six percent of them were identified to be nurses. Watson (2005) describes how medicine and technology are stripping nursing of its heart and soul. It's good to know that there are still nurses who reach out and go above and beyond the technical aspects of nursing. They "offer a ray of light in the institutional darkness of the patient's world." (Watson, 2005, p. 914)

Doty's Story:

"My experience is with a nurse in a doctor's office in Bloomington, IN. She and her actions left no doubt that she CARED! Her words and actions made me know she was giving her all to me."

This one says it all. Actions speak louder than words many times. "And be kind to one another, tenderhearted, forgiving one another, even as God in Christ forgave you." Ephesians 4:32 (*Life Application Study Bible*, NKJV, 1996)

Sissy's Story:

"I was taken to a local hospital six days after Hurricane Katrina with fever, vomiting and severe diarrhea. I stayed in the hospital for 5 days. On the third day I was diagnosed with salmonella from our well water—no fun! I was given only liquids and administered over 20 bags of IV [intravenous] fluids. There was no TV reception; the windows were boarded up—I think the hospital was being run by a generator. Not all doctors and nurses were able to be back at work due to the hurricane. The nurses and doctors that assisted me had their own storm related problems, but they treated me with kindness and were very personally concerned. I was pleased with their service—very unlike the help I received in the emergency room, but then that's another story!"

Despite the emotional distress the nurses were experiencing with their losses following the storm, they still displayed compassionate care to this patient during the immediate aftermath of the hurricane.

Anne's Stories:

"NOT LISTENING! Lots of nurses do not really listen. Usually they are checking medications and equipment, which I'm always thankful for. I've tried asking for a needle [IV catheter] in my hand to be checked because it really hurt. The nurse didn't listen or she ignored me. My hand started swelling and hurt more, but even though I complained again and asked for it to be looked at, I had to wait for the next shift 10 hours later! I don't remember what was wrong with the needle in my hand. But I will never forget the nurse!

That's the only bad experience I have had in nursing. I'm always extremely grateful for their care. Most of the questions I have after all surgeries I ask the nurse I have. They may not always answer the question, but they help keep you patient until the doctor comes.

I have been blessed many times with health care instructions, because they don't talk over my head to my husband and kids. I always want to know everything I should or should not do at home. Sometimes I see the doctor for check-out of the hospital, but most times it's just the nurse. Most nurses have enough patience to explain things to you more than once, if I just don't understand."

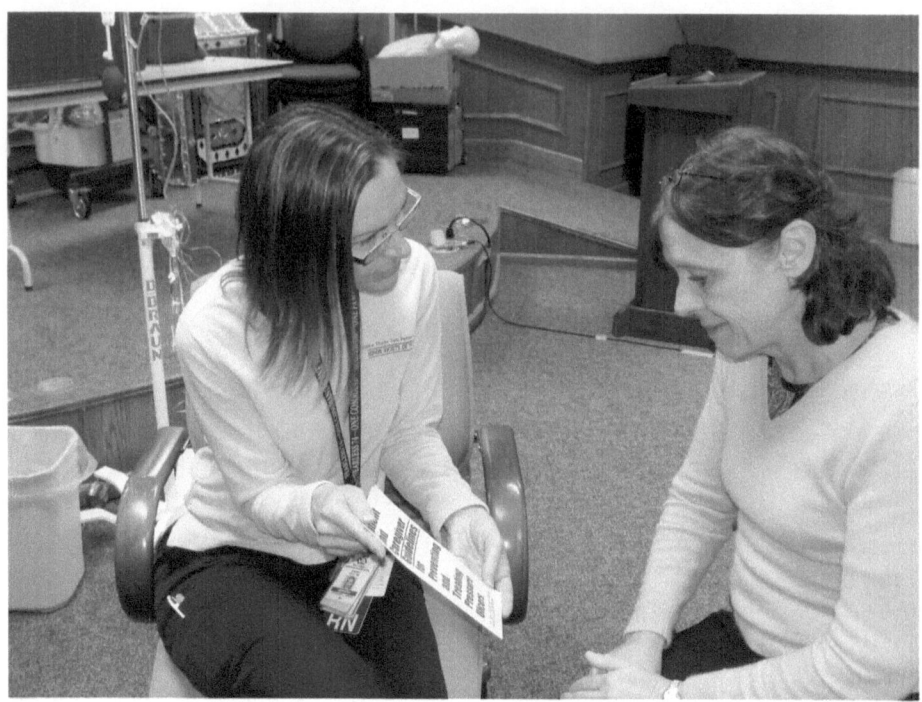

Anne describes several of the seven primary dimensions of patient-centered care. The first one she shares is the need to feel like she was being heard. In these days of nursing, and healthcare in general, listening to patients is neither expected nor compensated by healthcare agencies. Patients want their caregivers to be attentive and present. They want us to listen to them; don't just hear and walk away, but listen and interact with them. Let them know we are hearing them. To me, listening to someone is a passive action, but actually hearing what is being said is an active action. Sometimes it just takes repeating one thing that was said to confirm to the patient that he was heard. Listening falls under the very first dimension—respect for patient's values, preferences and expressed needs. Watson (2002) also describes the importance of listening with an open heart and compassion, without interruption, because it is a gift of one's self. It is healing.

A second dimension she describes is information, communication and education. She discusses that a patient likes it when the nurses and physicians spend that extra time explaining what he should expect, and what to do after discharge. This leads into the third and fourth dimensions of care. Those are 1) transition and continuity of care and

2) involving family and friends in the decision making process and encouraging their support.

She also discussed a fifth dimension which was physical comfort. This is the only dimension she mentioned that had a negative comment regarding nursing. Her IV site was apparently infiltrated and causing her pain, but the responses she got from the nursing staff were neither desirable nor acceptable. The one thing she said that pretty much summed it up regarding this was, "I don't remember what was wrong with the needle in my hand. But I will *never* (my emphasis) forget the nurse!"

A second story submitted by Anne follows: "My mother was in ICU after having surgery because of a brain aneurysm. My husband and I stayed there, because we knew she wouldn't be going home. I can never write enough praise for the nurses that took care of my mother. There was more sympathy and compassion that we ever expected. But there was one person there that I can never tell how much she meant to me and my mother. When we couldn't talk a lot we could look at each other and even that helped more than she knows."

This story describes a sixth dimension of patient-centered care—emotional support and alleviations of anxiety and fear. Involvement of family and friends is described again as well.

Libby's Stories:

"It was New Year's Eve and I had a roommate. We got along real well. I was in the 6th grade and was about 12 years old. I had a ligament transplant from my leg to my arm because of Erb's palsy [brachial plexus injury from birth]. A nurse ordered pizza and ice cream, and bought some party poppers to play with. He made it very fun. It was hilarious." [Libby's mother shared a more recent experience]: "In 2005, she had to have tendons released in her fingers of her affected hand. Following the surgery, she got very sick with nausea and vomiting. The nurses checked on her frequently and were very compassionate. They acted like they really loved their jobs."

This is an example of going that extra step—above and beyond—to make an unpleasant situation for children (being in a hospital) be more tolerable at a time that is usually promoted as "party time!" Libby's mom talks about how the nurses were compassionate and loved their jobs—again, loving and caring equals compassion!

Joan's Story:

"When my mother-in-law and my aunt were in the nursing home, there were some nurses that cared. Others were very rude to my aunt. I would bring supper on Friday night from a restaurant because they liked fish. But because my aunt would not eat what they cooked there (loaded with onions), they would not let me bring it to her. She was in her right mind too. She gradually got skinny and I could have cried. Then I saw a lady across the hall from my mother-in-law. Because she could not get out of her wheelchair, she would wet the chair; she could not help it. They would make her sleep on a cold plastic mattress without sheets, and she would take newspapers from the lobby to her room (hid them in her wheelchair) and lay them on her bed at night. She said it was so cold; so I went in one morning and I put sheets on her bed from my mother-in-law's room (they were going to change her bed later). The aide came over to me and asked did I see who had put the sheets on; I said I did. She said, "Well I took them off and don't put any more on because she wets herself on purpose just to get back at us." I said I did not believe this. She developed pneumonia and stayed in [a local hospital] for 2 weeks. She was hooked up to all kinds of machines and died 2 weeks later. She had no family at all. But let me tell you something, they are going to pay one day. My sister-in-law turned them in and the lady at the desk came to my mother-in-law's room and told her she didn't care if she did turn her in. After that my mother-in-law started (so called) falling out of her wheelchair and would be bruised all over her hips and arms. My sister-in-law had her transferred to another city. There she stayed (wet) every time we went so they moved her to a personal care home that was run by an elderly woman (little country lady). They were so sweet to her; she passed there."

This is a negative story shared by Joan which describes inattentive care; one of the things mentioned by respondents in the Gerteis, et al (1993) book regarding being cared for by competent caregivers. Another important requirement identified in that national survey was that they expected the provision of basic nursing care. This basic care includes maintaining normal body functions and providing a supportive atmosphere for healing and recuperation. The attitudes portrayed in this story certainly depict neglectful care, but also despiteful care. I pray this is not a common occurrence.

Marian's Story:

"Both of my parents passed away while on hospice services, at home. While I was already a nurse at the time, I was a new grad for the first death, and I still did not understand death and dying, or patient's rights when it came to this issue. With the help of a caring hospice team, I not only grew personally, but professionally. I am a big hospice advocate to this day."

A lot of the research I reviewed was done related to the care of hospice and oncology patients. Radwin, Farquar, Knowles and Virchick (2005) did a qualitative research of cancer patients' descriptions of their nurses' care. They ended up with four categories: 1) laudable [praiseworthy], defined as commendable qualities of the nurse and nursing care, 2) caring, defined as showing compassion, concern and kindness, 3) professional, defined as meeting expected standards of knowledge, skill, and demeanor, and 4) outcomes, defined as affective, cognitive, or physical effects attributed to nursing care. There were positive and negative comments obtained. The category that received the largest number of data was laudable (commendable qualities), second, was caring, third, professional, and fourth, outcomes. There were 461 patients who answered the questionnaire. As identified in this study, outcomes are not that important to patients. How they are treated—with commendable nursing care, by nurses who are compassionate and caring and exhibit their knowledge and competence—that's what is important to people.

Mark's Story:

"The nurse I felt was most compassionate *stopped* what she was doing—looked you in the eye and *actually* listened. You could *feel* the compassion. When we left she actually cried. You can tell the nurses that have a 'true calling.'"

Jean Watson (1999) is a nursing theorist and she believes that nurses become nurses because it is part of their being. They are "called" into the caring-healing profession. She believes that it is "love . . . or humanity itself which brings nurses into nursing and must be sustained if nursing and human caring is to survive." (Watson, 2005, p. 914).

I experienced this love and caring-healing professionalism personally when another one of my aunts was in ICU following surgery to repair a ruptured brain aneurysm. She did well right after surgery. But her blood pressure was too high and she eventually had a massive stroke. After a few days, the doctors finally told her children that she was brain dead and the only thing keeping her alive was the ventilator. After making the agonizing decision to stop the ventilator, the family wanted to be with her as much as possible. My aunt had five children ranging in ages from the 20s to the 50s, many grandchildren and great grandchildren, plus sisters, nieces, nephews and her mother (my grandmother). The visiting hours were 20 minutes at 5:00 am, 9:00 am, 12:00 pm and 9:00 pm, then two hours from 3:00 to 5:00 pm. The family had been in the waiting room coming and going for days prior to this, but the extended family let her immediate family members go back during visiting times. Some of my extended family really wanted to see her and talk to her, so I talked to her nurse, Peggy. She was so compassionate and caring, that once she made arrangements with the rest of the staff and explained to all the other patients, she allowed each and every one of us—two by two—to visit in her room, hold her hand, talk to her, and say our good-byes. I went back there with several of my family members, including my grandmother, who had already lost one daughter and now was out-living her oldest daughter. It was a very emotional time, and I will never forget how wonderful Peggy was to us. She stayed close by in case we needed anything, but let us grieve as a family.

Another memory I have is when my mother-in-law was in the ICU for about a week when one of the doctors decided to quickly remove her from the ventilator. He didn't wean her off; he just pulled the tube out to see how she would do. After about three hours, between her anxiety and pain, she was unable to breathe deeply enough to adequately keep her lungs working effectively, so she stopped breathing. Since I had been a nurse for over 25 years at that time, I expected that was going to happen. I had observed how she was wearing out while I was visiting with her, so I did what I could to prepare my family for what might happen. I was very upset and frightened, and when I heard the operator announce the "code" that someone had stopped breathing or his heart had stopped beating, I just knew it was her! Sure enough, it was. While the response team worked on her, a friend of mine came to the hall where the family was waiting. Pam offered comforting words, and then did one of the most important things she could do at that time to help our family. She offered to pray with us. She took us into a private room, and prayed a beautiful prayer to Jesus that lifted our spirits. Once they got her re-connected to the ventilator, we were allowed back to her room to visit her. She was awake and alert.

The Lord allowed us to have a few more days with her before He decided to take her to be with Him. When that happened, another nurse, Bill, allowed every one of the family members who had been in the waiting room when she died (which was about 20 people) to go into the room, as he prayed while we held hands around her. It was like having a worship service in the presence of the Lord.

CHAPTER 5

Examples of Compassion Found in the Bible:

Probably one of the most well-known stories people have heard or read is the story of the Good Samaritan. Jesus told this parable to his disciples about a man who was attacked by thieves, beaten and left half dead. A priest and a Levite came upon the man, but passed by him on the other side of the road. Finally a Samaritan man came across him and felt compassion for him. He bandaged him, put him on his donkey and took him to an inn where he took care of him. This describes compassion in action—the Samaritan recognized the distress of the beaten man and did something about it.

In the Old Testament, there are several examples of compassion. In Exodus 2, verse 6 the story of the Pharaoh's daughter when she found the baby, Moses, in a basket floating in the river is described. "And when she opened it, she saw the child, and behold, the baby wept. So she had *compassion* on him, and said, 'This is one of the Hebrew's children.'" If she had not had compassion on him, Moses may have been left to die or may not have grown up to lead the Hebrew children out of bondage to the Egyptians.

Elisha, the prophet, showed *compassion* on the widow woman whose creditors were threatening to take her two sons to pay her debt. He tells her to take her only possession of one jar of oil and to gather as many empty vessels from neighbors that she could borrow. Then she was to pour her jar of oil into each empty vessel until they were full. When all the vessels were full, she asked her sons for another one and there were none—then there was no more oil. She took the oil and sold it to pay her debt.

Another example is when Elisha was given his own room to stay when he would go through the Shunammite woman's town. She had *compassion* on him as he travelled, and she had her husband build a special room for him to stay in. Later, the Shunammite woman's son became ill and died in her lap while she was waiting on Elisha to come to her. Elisha demonstrated *compassion* when he arrived and covered the child's body until it became warm again, and the child was healed by God. (2 Kings 4:8-37)

Everyone is familiar with the story of Jonah being thrown into the sea because he was running from God, and a huge storm was causing the boat he was on to almost wreck. Prior to the men throwing him overboard, they had *compassion* for him and tried to out-row the storm. "And he [Jonah] said to them, 'Pick me up and throw me into the sea; then the sea will become calm for you. For I know that this great tempest is because of me.' Nevertheless the men rowed hard to return to land, but they could not, for the sea continued to grow more tempestuous against them." (Jonah 1:12-13)

There are multiple examples of when Jesus showed compassion. In Matthew, chapter 9, verse 36 it states, "But when He saw the multitudes, He was moved with *compassion* for them, because they were weary and scattered, like sheep having no shepherd." And in chapter 14, verse 14 it says, "And when Jesus went out He saw a great multitude; and He was moved with *compassion* for them and healed their sick."

In the book of Mark, we find the story of when Jesus showed *compassion* for the paralytic man whose four friends lifted him to the roof of the building Jesus was in, and broke through the roof to get him to Jesus. Jesus healed him for his faith. (Mark 2:3-5) The story of one of the rulers of the synagogue named Jarius who requested Jesus to heal his 12 year old daughter who was near death. Jesus had *compassion* on Jarius and followed him to his home where the child had already died. He raised her from death and instructed her parents to not tell anyone what had happened, but to feed their daughter. (Mark 5:22-24, 35-43)

Another well-known story is the parable Jesus told of the "prodigal son" in Luke 15, verses 11-22. The youngest son of a man asked for his share of his father's income to be given to him, and then he left his father's home. The boy squandered the money and ended up working on a pig farm wishing he could have what the pigs were eating. He decided to go back to his father's house and ask him to let him be a servant, but his father saw him from afar and had *compassion* on him. He ran to meet him and welcome him back home.

In John, chapter 8 and verses 2-11, is the story of the woman who was caught in adultery and was confronted by scribes and Pharisees. They threatened to stone her to death as that was what had been commanded by Moses in the Old Testament. Jesus instructed them that the one who did not have sin in his life should be the one to throw the first stone. They all left the woman and Jesus by themselves. Jesus was showing *compassion* towards the woman by keeping her from being stoned to death.

In an anonymous pastor's sermon posted on the world wide web, he describes God's great compassion. The difference between us and

God is that God has an infinite supply of mercy, compassion and love to give to all of us on a daily basis. If we are in His will, doing what He desires us to do, we will have an abundant, unending supply, as well, through Him, because in Luke, chapter 6, verse 38, Jesus says, "Give and it will be given to you: . . . For with the same measure that you use, it will be measured back to you." The more compassion one demonstrates to patients and family, the more respect they will have for a nurse who spends the few extra minutes with them—that's usually all it takes.

God has compassion not only on *lifetime problems* like illnesses, nor only on *eternal promises* like redemption, but He has compassion for our *daily needs* as well. It would serve nurses well to remember that and remember to take care of the patient holistically. But many times, nurses tend to focus on the daily needs (physical) without looking at the lifetime (family) needs or eternal (spiritual) needs.

So should nurses have compassion? Absolutely, there should be compassion demonstrated in nursing. However, there are times that the nurse needs compassion and understanding. There may be days that the nurse has been dealing with death and dying, critical illness and chronic illness so much that it is easier to just "do her job" by completing the tasks that need to be done and just go home. It isn't necessarily because the nurse isn't compassionate, but that she is fatigued from the endless hours of caring for the sick. Hopefully, this book will give nurses a reminder that we are in this business to take care of people when they are ill and sometimes that means they are dying. But on the other hand, people in the community will have a better understanding of nursing and give them ideas of the daily stressors that can be encountered in nursing.

APPENDIX A

Name: (optional) _____ Date: _____
Contact information: (optional) _____

Gender: _____ Male _____ Female
Age: _____ 18-24 _____ 40-49 _____ 70-79
_____ 25-30 _____ 50-59 _____ > 80
_____ 31-39 _____ 60-69 _____ Other _____

1) Have you ever been in any of the following as a patient? (choose all that apply)
   a) Hospital
   b) Nursing home
   c) Your home
   d) Rehab center

2) Has anyone in your family been in any of the following as a patient? (choose all that apply)
   a) Hospital
   b) Nursing home
   c) Your home
   d) Rehab center

3) Has anyone you know other than family been in any of the following as a patient? (choose all that apply)
   a) Hospital
   b) Nursing home
   c) Your home
   d) Rehab center

4) How would you define the word compassion? (match the letters to the words)
   a) Sharing of another's feelings, experiences, and emotions.
   b) The state of being cruel or barbarous.

c) Concern for another's suffering or misfortune combined with a desire to help.
d) Concern for another's feelings, experiences, and emotions.
_____ compassion
_____ empathy
_____ hostility
_____ sympathy

5) Using the definition of compassion as "Feeling concerned about other's suffering and having a desire to ease the suffering," answer the following question: In your experience(s), how would you rate (from 1-7) the level of compassion of the nurses caring for you or your loved one or friend? (circle one)
1 = no compassion at all 7 = demonstrated great compassion

1 2 3 4 5 6 7

6) In your opinion, which of the following indicate(s) that a nurse is compassionate(circle all that apply)?
a) Plans quality time with the patient f) Problem solves to resolve patient concerns
b) Actively listens to the patient g) Involves patient in the plan of care
c) Always presents with a caring attitude h) Involves the family in the plan of care when can
d) Keeps promises i) Provides dignity and respect to patient/ family
e) Keeps patient informed of changes

7) Write an example to explain the above 2 answers (as many words or pages at it takes). You may give as many examples as you wish.

Date received: _____

REFERENCES

Abendroth, M. & Flannery, J. (2006). Predicting the risk of compassion fatigue: A study of hospice nurses. *Journal of Hospice and Palliative Nursing. 8*(6), 346-356.

Alkema, K., Linton, J. M., & Davies, R. (2008). A study of the relationship between self-care, compassion satisfaction, compassion fatigue, and burnout among hospice professionals. *Journal of Social Work in End-of-Life and Palliative Care, 4* (2), 101-119.

Aycock, N. & Boyle, D. (2009) Interventions to manage compassion fatigue in oncology nursing. *Clinical Journal of Oncology Nursing 13* (2), 183-191.

Davidson, J. E. (2009). Family-centered care: Meeting the needs of patients' families and helping families adapt to critical illness. *Critical Care Nurse, 29* (3), 28-34. AACN Critical Care Journals.

Drane, J. F. (2002). Honesty in medicine. *http://www.bioetica.uchile.cl/ doc/ honesty.htm.*

Gerteis, M, Edgman-Levitan, S, Daley, J., & Delbanco, T.L. (Eds) 1993. *Through the patient's eyes: Understanding and promoting patient-centered care.* Jossey-Bass Publishers: San Francisco.

Life Application Study Bible, New King James Version (1996). Tyndale House Publishers: Wheaton, IL.

Lama, XIV, D. 2005. *The Power of Compassion: A Collection of Lectures.* (translated by Geshe Thupten Jinpa). Thorsons: London.

Laschinger, H.K.S., Leiter, M.P. May, 2006. The impact of nursing work environments on patient safety outcomes: The mediating role of burnout/engagement. *The Journal of Nursing Administration, 36* (5), 259-267.

Radwin, L.E., Farquhar, S.L., Knowles, M. N., & Virchick, B. G. (2005). Cancer patients' descriptions of their nursing care. *Journal of Advance Nursing 50* (2), 162-169.

Rohan, E. & Bausch, J. (2009). Climbing Everest: Oncology work as an expedition in caring. *Journal of Psychosocial Oncology. 27*(1), 84-118.

Schultz, PR. October, 1987. When client means more than one: Extending the foundational concept of person. *Advances in Nursing Science,* Aspen Publishers, Inc; 10(1), 71-86.

Swanson, K. M. (1990). Providing care in the NICU: Sometimes an act of love. *Advances in Nursing Science 13* (1), 60-73. Aspen Publishers, Inc.

The American Heritage® Dictionary of the English Language, Fourth Edition copyright ©2000 by Houghton Mifflin Company. Updated in 2009. Published by *Houghton Mifflin Company.*

Townsend, J. 2007. *Loving people: How to love and be loved.* Thomas Nelson Publishers: Nashville.

Watson, J. 1999. *Postmodern nursing and beyond.* Churchill Livingstone, Edinburgh.

Watson, J. (2002). Love and caring: Ethics of face and hand—an invitation to return to the heart and soul of nursing and our deep humanity. *Nursing Administrative Quarterly.* (July—September), 197-202.

Watson, J. (2005). Guest editorial: What, may I ask is happening to nursing knowledge and professional practices? What is nursing thinking at this turn in human history? *Journal of Clinical Nursing,* **14**, 913-914.

www.ingramcontent.com/pod-product-compliance
Lightning Source LLC
Chambersburg PA
CBHW050344290526
45785CB00006B/2623